The Things Between Us

The Things Between Us
Living Words: Anthology 1

Words and poems of people experiencing dementia

Shoving Leopard

Shoving Leopard
100/8 Great Junction Street,
Edinburgh, EH6 5LD
United Kingdom

https://www.facebook.com/ShovingLeopard

First published in 2014

The Things Between Us;
Living Words: Anthology 1
www.livingwords.org.uk
info@livingwords.org.uk
07967 502506

ISBN 978-1-905565-24-5

This anthology
is dedicated to all the people
Living Words has met and worked with
between 2007 and 2014.

Contents

Forewords

To read the poems in Living Words is like dipping into a basin of water, and trying to hold the droplets in your hands as you splash your face with pure joy. So many memories are triggered through these precious words, from so many folk going through their own private and personal musings. We all know the frustration of trying to find that word on the tip of the tongue. Imagine what it feels like to search for the face of a loved one? To try and grasp that once familiar feeling when you see a face you nearly recognise? Imagine looking into a mirror and asking "Who is this?" Tracing the lines on the skin and wondering where all the years have gone?

Living Words helps to ease the pain and share the joy of things remembered. It is an anthology to dip into like a box of chocolates. I would so love to have had this book when my mother was struggling with Alzheimer's. I know she would have been able to catch a moment here and there. One of the hardest things to deal with as a Carer was the repetition of conversation. I would get irritated and would feel so guilty. What better way to communicate when conversation dries up than through the words of others who are in the same place?

I have always said that we can all deal with the big stuff when it hits, but it is the flipping minutiae of life that gets you down. Not so the poems in this anthology, it turns the minute observations into huge pearls of wisdom to help us all get through the day. Enjoy!

Lynda Bellingham
17th March 2014

It does not happen very often that we are invited into a person's life and find something hidden, like discovering a secret door that could conceal a long, softly lit corridor. At the end of the corridor there might be spiral stairs, which take us aloft to a circular room, leading to a square room and then another room of an undeterminable shape opening up onto a courtyard where we are greeted by all of humanity's feelings, memories, dreams, frustrations, aspirations, fears and loves. *The Things Between Us* delivers rays of sunlight into the courtyard of dementia as all of us—people with a dementia, carers, families, healthcare staff, artists, academics, community members—encounter and experience this confusing and unwelcome syndrome of symptoms and behaviours we have come to label as dementia.

This important anthology reminds us that above all else, there is a human being caught up in a tremendous change to their lives, a change that they did not invite, a change that is taking them, their families and friends, carers and all who know them, down different secret corridors each day.

In his poem *Ithaka*, the Greek-born Egyptian poet C.P. Cavafy, describing a life's journey, writes of the dangerous Laistrygonians, Cyclops and angry Poseidon but cautions us, "don't be afraid of them: you'll never find things like that on your way as long as you keep your thoughts raised high, as long as a rare excitement stirs your spirit and your body." The syndrome of dementia throws many extreme cognitive, emotional and behavioural challenges into people's lives but the poetry contained in *The Things Between Us* reminds us, both joyfully and painfully, like the good poetry it is, that people with a dementia have a lot to say—and they want to say it—but the rest of us need to listen and if we can take the time to do so, we too may discover a rare excitement that stirs our spirits and our bodies.

In closing, it seems to me that we might be paying too much attention to the symptoms of the different dementias and not nearly enough attention to how the arts might contribute to rehabilitation for people with a dementia. I would urge Health and Wellbeing Boards, Clinical Commissioning Groups, NHS memory clinics, social care services and charities, along with the rest of us, to please listen and consider how poetry and other art forms can positively impact the wellbeing and quality of life of those with a dementia and the people who care for them. Some of that evidence is contained right here.

Paul M. Camic, FRSPH
Professor of Psychology & Public Health
Salomons Centre for Applied Psychology
Canterbury Christ Church University
18th March 2014

Introduction

Welcome to Living Words' first anthology, *The Things Between Us*. Inside these pages you will find the words and poems of individuals we have worked with between autumn 2007 and January 2014. All the participants are experiencing a dementia and live in UK care homes. These insightful, moving and surprising pieces represent thousands of words and poems crafted during that time and are a drop in the ocean of the lives being lived inside the silent margins of UK society today. For a variety of reasons the names of the contributors are not included in this publication - their words have to speak for them. As you dip in and out of these words I invite you to take a moment to give them acknowledgment and thanks.

About Living Words

Living Words began working with people experiencing a dementia in 2007. Since then we have conducted residencies in care homes, nursing homes, community settings, arts centres and hospitals. At the start it was just me, following my nose, discovering what this work would be with the intention of communicating in the moment using silence, the spoken and written word. What emerged has been honed over the years into a methodology, a person-centred approach and programme that we want to see taking place across the UK and beyond.

The first person I worked with was in a hospital in London. At the end of our four weeks of working together, she took my hands, looked deep into my eyes and said: "Now you know two worlds – the one outside and the one inside, in me. And you've got to go and tell all the people." This has been Living Words' mission ever since. The residencies inspire our wider programme of performances and publications. We aim to share the inside world of people whose voices are not usually heard, so that together we can all learn to see the person not the diagnosis, and so face dementia head on.

Living Words residencies are now a five stage programme:

1) Working one-to-one with individuals experiencing a dementia to create their own Living Words Word Books. This is the main part of the programme.

2) Working one-to-one with staff. In the same way that we work with residents we work with a small number of staff, so that they experience what the residents have been experiencing. We strongly support carers in our work.

3) Every participant receives their own Living Words Word Book. They are given out and read with individuals. We hold staff workshops, looking at the words participants have spoken and how these words might affect daily practice; we look at how to use the books as a communication bridge.

4) Staff commit to a 'project'. This aims to embed the books and communication techniques from the workshop.

5) A sharing event is held. Staff, residents and relatives come together. Words and poems are shared, staff read and talk about using the books and they receive certificates.

In becoming a charity we look forward to gaining the funding and support required to enable many more people to experience Living Words.

Listening

The art of listening is crucial to our work. We listen with open, blank minds. Through eye contact and quality of attention, we enter into the "shared experience" with participants. Trainer, therapist and colleague Danuta Lipinska says of this: "Within the myriad realms of silence... I imagine it akin to a prism being held aloft between us." [1] Physically between the two of you is the book and pen, ready to write down and validate the words expressed. Sometimes we sit in silence for a while, other times words come quickly. We do not judge or try to "make sense" of what a person is saying.

Several years ago a woman said to me: "You listen at a different level, cos it's happening at a different level." This listening requires a lot of trust in yourself and the process. You have to stay listening when you are going against convention and "normal" conversation. You have to go to that other level – and through listening "behind the words" you, as listener, are able to know the significance of words. Through listening on that "other level" the words that a person speaks are poetry. Listen and you hear the poet speak.

Living Words Word Books

The words of each individual are put into sections. In collaboration with each person we read them back their own words as we edit, and their response becomes the title. The words are laid on the page to be read out loud.

Each participant chooses a front cover image and is presented with their Word Book. We work with staff on how to use the book as a communication bridge. The focus is on connecting through reading a person's words aloud. The focus is not on getting to the end of a poem or the whole book.

When a person hears their words back they often do not recall having said the words, or who they spoke the words to. But they feel the resonance of their words and often respond with: "Yes," "That's it," "So true," or: "That sounds like me." A person's sense of well-being and personhood is elevated.

People have used their Word Book to show doctors how they feel, or they keep it on their person at all times as if to say: "Look. I am still worth something – this book shows that." I once returned to a home I had not been to for a while and a woman I had previously worked with introduced herself as a poet and showed me her Word Book.

About this anthology
Choosing which poems to include has been a tough job - we could have filled at least twenty books. In a way these poems have chosen themselves. Though some of these sections and words might appear sad or "depressing", they represent the reality of a person's experience. Yes, when read aloud with the individual they are sometimes met with tears - but tears of *relief*. A person can experience a hiatus from the feelings of confusion, inadequacy and loss.

We hope you are able to take a lot from this collection and we look forward to welcoming you to one of our performances or events as we give platform to the living words of people whose lives and experiences remain hidden. Thank you very much.

Susanna Howard
Founder and Artistic Director, Living Words
18th March 2014

[1] Danuta Lipinska, *Person-Centred Counselling for People with Dementia: Making Sense of Self*, (Jessica Kingsley, 2009)

THINKING

'Pulled it all from the cellar'

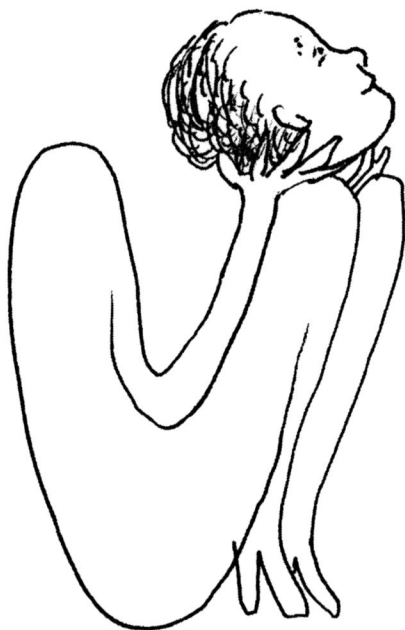

Think

I don't know what I think
I don't know if it matters
I don't think it does
I don't think
I don't know that I think
That's the trouble

Want People To Know What It's Like

I'm thinking about eggs
And she's talking about work
As if everything is the same but it ain't
Everything and everyone is different
Everybody don't sink the same
Or feel the same.
You can listen to everything and
Not listen a word they say
I can't make it right
We all think we're different
Not think of anybody else
Listen, I'm thinking about eggs

What Is? What Are? What?

You must see a lot of characters
In here we all think so differently
Yet along the same lines

So many people aren't there
So many different thoughts flying around
Don't know which to gather in

Do you do much thinking or daydreaming?
We all dream different things
It's interpretation, that's the point
What one does with them
People, fascinating

That's Somebody

That's somebody
Walking around
With high heels on

I think I've given you
Nothing very special
Don't think
Can't think
Of anything else
But I am -
I don't know anymore

There's people
Going back and forth
There's not much I can do
That's somebody
Going back and forth
Walking around

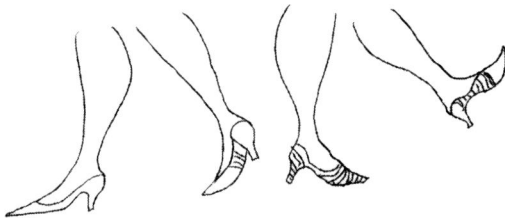

Words From The Cellar

I'm finding myself such a quick way
Been dealing with and
Telling them you definitely
Gonna get stuff
From the cellar
But now, don't work -
Pulled it all from the cellar
And you were left and so was I
Gone, all gone

All Of Us

Why do we make ourselves worry
About others?
Why worry?
Why rushing for?
Why running for?
You don't stop and think
Do we?
I don't know why or where or what
I been doing
I'm just rocking out
Through me bits

Slowly

I don't know much
It just comes up, half bits, sort of thing
You know you can't think
That's what it is
Here with this croaky like, can't speak
Slowly, can't think anymore

Ticking

After you've gone, it's quiet
But my brain is still going.
I speak my mind, my feeling
It comes naturally -
Everybody can have it,
Anybody can have it -
You are human person, that is all.

My brain is still ticking -
Is very ordinary, common.
My brain is still warm -
Inquisitive
Turn the page,
Put the reader in it
Not all me, me, me.

After you've gone, it's quiet
But my brain is still working
Still going
Still ticking
Still warm

Can't Think

I can't think
Can't think of what you're thinking
I don't know, was thinking
Of getting back, back to what?
Can't see anything
Don't know what to do
I'm frightened I'm going to
Go again, I've been frightened -
This is my gaga
Oh blimey
I'm alright
Love being here with you
Don't know what to do

Machines

Some people have machines –
They don't run on.
Others don't.

Sometimes it is overused
Sometimes doesn't even need reminding.
Hardly going to control it again.

You think it lies with one person
But discover it lies with others -
Because that's the part
The world is different.

Some people have machines
Sometimes overused
Others don't.

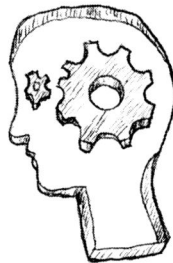

Pictures

I got pictures
Go in my mind all the time -
Went to church twelve and carried on
Perhaps I was wrong -
Should have done something?
Haven't done anything really.
Things go through my mind
And I can't think of anything

Not Too Bad Really

Trying to think of my own name
All you can say really, it's ridiculous
Sorry about this - I'm trying to think
What have we got round the corner?

Ridiculous not to be aware of
What I should be doing. Just can't
Get my mind fixed to it, try
And get my mind to it, together

Things worry me a bit
To be perfectly honest -
Can't pull anything
Out of the bag

The Back Doorstep

Two or three clever things
In the back of my mind
Unfortunately
They seem to stick
To the back of my mind -
You don't do them.
That expression 'back of my mind'
Really rather significant:
You forget it's a phrase
And doesn't state that you
Are scrubbing the back doorstep

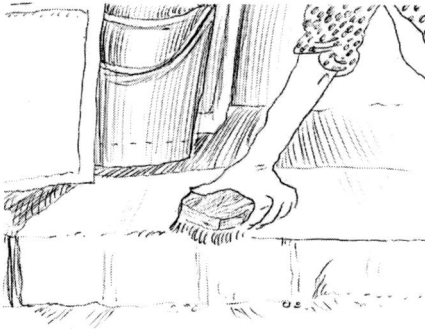

Coming Back

The self is coming back
Sometimes, to what it was
Don't even know if you're
Going or coming, sometimes
The head don't serve me
As it should, tough sometimes
But I'm a survivor
But don't remember nothing
Sometimes you have to think
Of what you have to do
Not alone
Everybody is thinking that

BOREDOM

'I'm sitting waiting, for what?'

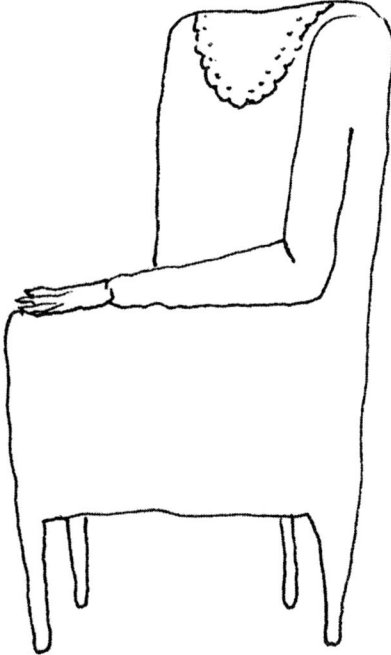

Lost

I don't know really, because
I'm really
Lost.

It scares me to hell
I don't know what to do -
I'm scared

It was so disgusting – I just sat there, doing
Nothing.
I thought I was
In an asylum I was
Ashamed that I
Sit there

These people were people who, well they are
Old age pensioners. They made me an
Old
Age
Pensioner. I was
Really annoyed - terrible isn't it

There's nothing wrong with me -
I just don't do
Anything.

I feel
Lost – that's all I can say, because
I've never felt
Lost - this is
Just hell

So you now have the whole thing. You've
Been told by me, from us going.
I can't say it myself.
The saddest thing.

Static

It's a funny old day
Not hot, not cold, not warm
It's static
Breathing's my trouble
That's why I'm here
You look at that tree, not a leaf moving
I'm sitting here I can see it
In bed I can see it
Everything is static

How can I explain it?
Today is very dull
No life is going on
My breathing's a bit, take no notice
It's absolutely static
Not a leaf moving, ah!
It's moving now, make me out a liar
Just a little breeze
The tree is moving

The Things Between Us

These are the things between us:
We all day sit
Time on our hands
People have condition
People inclined to leave them alone
Feel loneliness
These are the things between us:
Open hearts, Open the door
The door of friendship
Life and everything

Again Moments

I've been shaking
My eyes are aching
Arms have gone funny again
Not steady on my feet
Have to be careful and
Mind my ps and qs
Have to squint at times
Can see the clock
But can't tell the time
It's moments I have
One minute on top
Yesterday under the weather
But now I feel alright
Got that under the collar feel
Hot, terrible, nervous, frightening
Feel funny, just stuck me
In the corridor -
Stew in me own blood

You Show Side, So Many Of Us - Asleep

All of us sleep in this house
It's better than the others
Having a sleep, a rest
Have a rest

They're having a sleep
Then they're gone
It's hard, sitting in a chair
Can't go to bed, bed
Oh our beds! Why?

They're nearly all
Going to sleep
In the house – right! All!
So bad
Because they see you
And change you
And go to sleep

Do you feel sad
To write it down?
There's no life
I'm tired
I can't lay down

I'm In Bed

Such a lovely day - should be out
Normally - I'm an active person
There's nowhere to go.
What is important to me is
To get up and get out.

Every day of my life I get up, out
Even if I have things to do
Now I miss it very much
Trouble is if you are not well
God help you! The worst thing in life

If not well and not capable
Have to be a certain type of person
I'm not that kind
Between you and me, I like to get up
But I'm just lying down here
Waiting to see what will happen

It Is Too

Only thing is I cannot talk, you know
It goes the wrong way – awful.
It's not me, I was very active

You see I don't know a lot of women here
So I sit and try and breathe to myself
Or go to sleep

In here, some of them I went to school with
They sit there day after day, nothing for them
You have to sit there and look, it's all
I was never up for that, no –
Like sitting on hot stone

I See Something

I see something
Thought I saw something
Looked like sunshine
That's what nature does
Cause confusion in all directions –
Never lets you know.
Nice things are growing
At least we'll have something to look at:
We don't reckon on a great deal of
Sunshine or warmth or fun and games.

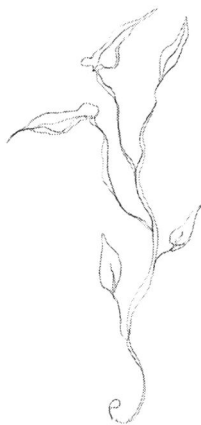

Don't Like Hanging About

Maybe it's best talking -
Made me in to a student
People are reasonable about it.
You're attacked by it,
Not very comfortable -
I don't know where to put myself.
On a bar to some extent,
I don't like hanging about

Life, it's upside down
We've had it for ages
I'm altered now
Don't know anymore
My feeling is that I -
Am I a duverand? (some would say?)
What's your feeling?
Yes, it's upside down.

I'm An Okay

I'd like to get out
I must renew
Want to feel the opposite
I'm jealous of you
I'm waiting
I'm waiting
I don't understand it
I'm waiting -
Very hard for me
I cannot get out
I'm wasted.
Been stolen. Stolen, yes
I'm a sorry, I -
Got nobody
Nobody
I don't understand it
Got nobody -
Very hard for me
I can't get out -
In here I'm an okay
Want to talk
Listen. Listen to me -
What will you think of me now?

It Is Perfect

Always sitting here, on me bum, that's me
It's quite true, I'm frightened
To say anything generally.
Probably boredom I think
It's the responsibility
Cope. Difficult. So easy.
It's unusual to sit and do bugger all
That's the point, it's true
I'm so active normally
But these days I'm not
I sit in this chair and rot
Perfect end of a story
Sit here

Overflow

Well I'm watching the world
Go round at the moment
Arranging a contract
For me to spend my emotions
I've got a bin there
That will take the
Overflow

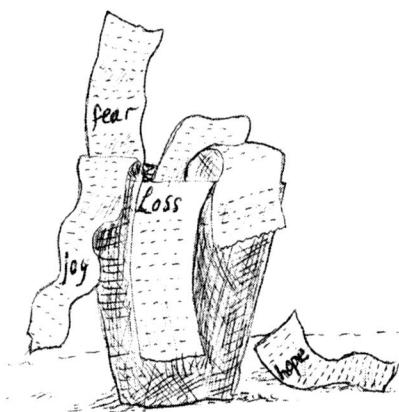

Now

What's for What?
I'm sitting, waiting, for what?
Nothing. Yes, I remember,
Don't know what it is, really
This waiting, for this
There's a lot of people here wanting things
I am needing something and you're
Here, right now
Right now
Right now
It will be done
Under the sun
And this is the
Best time
Cos we are now two, now two

☆

TIME

'You can't stop, can't clip it to'

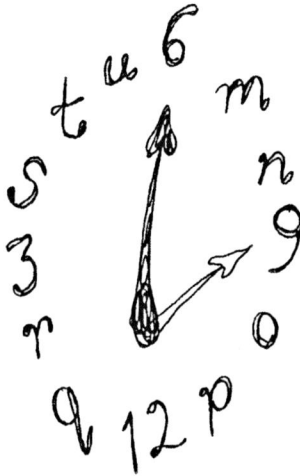

The Time Part

The time part -
It stands for everything
So you have to tell me something again
It is hard – the same thing for us all
You do not know again, again
This is what you suffer now
You have it all the time
You can't stop, can't clip it to
If everybody know and think
They can change it

Time Is So Ridiculous

What day are we on?
What are we doing at the moment?
What part of the year are we looking at?
I'm struggling now - feels fairly okay
Should be straight forward enough
What's the day did you say?
What part of the day is it?
Not taking things in

I have no trouble in sleeping
Just lie down and hope for the best
All you can do at the moment
Not much alternative

Come And Go

Don't take notice of me
If I look a bit crotchety
A nuisance when you
Wake up, under the weather
Hot, big sweats. Then it wears off.
And some mornings, up early
It's me feet, pains round ankle.
Comes and goes - 'You come and go'
A friend, she's always singing that
Linda, some time ago...
Feels better during the day
Comes and goes, here we go -
Don't like the ankle more than anything
Just when I wake up - Come and
Go, like everything else
Like I say – up and down
Like I say – comes and goes
Wake up feeling under weather
But haven't got me umbrella

In Today's Time

There are certain things I've been observing
Trying to find an answer
The world has been in existence for millions of years
Because we are here, we are part of history
And somebody reading your book will think why and what
They are only here for a moment
The book could be here for hundreds of years

Can't Come Out Of My Thoughts

So what must I think about you?
Watching me talk now
I feel nice, you are good
You remember -
Remember me all the time
But I'm telling you - you can't come out
Of my thoughts, I don't have the thought
Of a person -
I don't bring it up all the time
But I don't really remember
Me don't remember the time
Or the day
Get good remembrance sometime

On Writing

By the time you finish writing about me
And my whatever you call it
The number of sheets will be
Astronomical
How sure can one ever be?
What you are thinking and
What you are saying are
Two different things sometimes.
They were said by me at one time
How could I remember?
I get a funny feeling I forget things
When you think of it in one correct way
You realise I should have said it in
A different way to make me
Understand myself better
May not be valid
May be
That is how life is
It is something that happened during the some
time
Past time
Some time of time

What Am I Playing At?

I live in two places pretty well,
Trying to think on what the position is -
Why are we not playing the game we used to play?
Looking back I – What? I just can't think
I was more or less by myself
No longer in that position
I'll try, think, wait a minute...
How strange - in two positions, seem to be
My original thing all dates back
Cannot pull myself back
To what I have been.
Thinking back at the moment

Soon Goes The Time

I'm not in a hurry
We all join in together
You don't enjoy it when you get it
If you have a lot do you?
Time soon goes
Don't mind at all
I watch the people go
Come in and out and go
Soon be teatime
Some hopes, some hopes
Time goes too fast don't it
Got to stick to it, time
Soon goes
True
Does an' all

AGEING

'Whatever this is – has hit me'

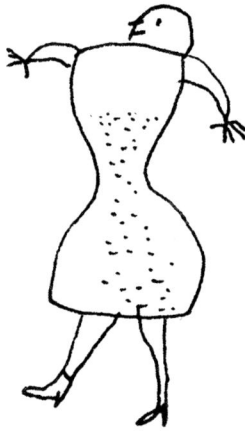

Up To Date

I'm 88
Which means the expression
'You've had it' is up to date -
Had most of what you're going to by then

I'm old and tired and a bit weary
I don't know what happened
And I miss my kids:
Better start thinking of the little bit
Left remaining -
My future.
I'm 88 years old
So I have a bit of explaining to do

Causes

Every now and again I get very emotional
Because I can't do thinks what I used to
Happens when you get old
Can remember some things
But because I've had a stroke
Can't remember all -
Didn't think I'd end up in a care home
Remember things that happened in the past
But today - like sometimes - I can't
And they still don't know what causes
Stroke

Seeing 1

Well I've got older haven't I
Suppose that's normal -
I'm not very good at writing
Can't see very well anymore
But I can see you and I can
Look at things and see things
But I don't know
What they're talking about
Cos I get mixed up - But I
Recognised you right away
Feels great, trust, talk
I'm getting older not dafter

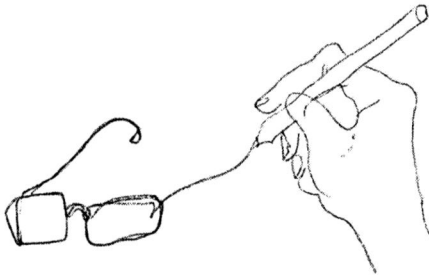

That's It

That's true
Don't forget, half a dozen umbrellas
That's enough
That's all
Don't lose your hat
That's what I'm saying
The snow will blow it away
That's good
That's it
I'm stuck at the window looking
That's it
That's it, again
Them words quick enough?
Have a read from top to bottom
I'll let you off
Is the end of the road
Portobello
That's it
That is it
I better not say anymore 'that's it'
Get old with every passing year
Older and older
That's it
No more 'that's it'
Getting to be a habit
That's it - see
Signed and sealed
Susanna does the writing
M does the notes
That's it
Oh no, that's it
'That's it' just comes
Naturally
Comes
That's it!

I Must Get My Teeth Done

I will
I must
Wanna get me teeth back
Today.
Got the money, get it done quick.

My hearing's not great and
I want my nails done and
I'm dying for a couple of tea,
Haven't had a cup of tea,
I'm dying, oh I hope not,
I'm trying to remember -
Shall we leave this place?
My teeth are bad
My face. It's gone.

Scream

A day old you were
'merp, merp, merp'
Couldn't write a word
But you could scream

The first breather of when born
A God send for the nurses
The mother
When they start to breathe
For themselves

Don't forget
When they come out of your belly
You've been doing all the work
For them
They do it for themselves
Terrific

Child birth is a miracle
I got two
Son and daughter
13 months between
First thing they did
Scream
Start breathing

All Embers

Old fashioned in't they
Sitting there
She wants to get up
They don't wanna do that do they
Some round here are all embers
That one's not thinking
He wants to remember it
Can he?
Now, see:
They've got habits

Day Centre

I'm a bit cut off here –
I got day centre, lovely there
There are five women we can ask for help
Always the same
Always know who you're talking to
So kind, lovely, beautiful.
Sometimes –
I would love to put a bed down there
Just be

We have a shop there, lovely
The woman comes to serve me and
I can't get it out
She laughs, says
'I think it's marmite is it?!'
It's true - all these little things

We had an idea the woman was going
And that was it –
We were all sort of in a state
Don't think I could bear it
If I couldn't go there
They've given some people notice
To pay money, to go there.
I don't have any money
So I wouldn't be able to go.

Good Time

What I might say
What I might do
Like to –
Go out and have a good old
You know
With me own
Oh how can I say?
Go out and have a
Oh gawd blimey, how can I say?
Go out and have
Somebody
My own age

That's what I mean
Have a good time

My Little Darling

2.
It's funny
I always wanted children
As I get older I feel it more and more
Go to the park in St John's Wood
Watch the little ones, I like that
It helps me 'cause it's too late for me
Now, to have children
An old woman
But my little darling, I like her
In my life

4.
To me she looks so real
My little baby
Poor little thing
Little nose, little chin

I get my pleasure from her
I look at her, makes me feel it's real
'You're my little darling'
Whoever made this doll
This face, quite an art
'I wish I had your face
People would fall in love with me'
I see her as real
She sits here all the time
I feel sorry for her
And that is what you are without children
Mad

8.
Do you think I'm mad?
People must think I'm mad
I feel, I wish, sometimes
These little dolls
Could talk to them and
They talk to you

9.
It's so important for women -
I feel as if I have really born her
I wash her every day
Like a human being
It is in me, I can't help it, love

Don't Get Old

Life is so difficult in this world
It would be nice to be
Where there was a little bit of cold
When you get older if you've got
The right people, it's alright.

You don't know whether it's yes or coming
Can't go out unless somebody took you

I pray to God to take me now
Might as well go – dead, to God
Not used to it, nothing in my life
Had a wonderful husband and he died
My eyes have gone bad, very sore
Might as well go on my own way
Be better to go to my husband

Whatever This Is

When it started off it was
Shocking to me, they'd say I said
Something and I'd not know, and now
Here I am at 96, is it 96?
What's this year?

I'm very old now
Whatever this is - has hit me
Will not get better at my age
It came on all of a sudden
Did notice different things I was doing
Funny things, sudden

Toffees

They were getting old, into the third act –
Near the end of it -
The bit where they do this
The girls, all in their night clothing
Their parents nearly worn out
Some can't go anywhere
It's a bit cracking
Be careful
They don't get many of the population you know
They double it up
They always have toffees

PEOPLE

'You're witness to what was'

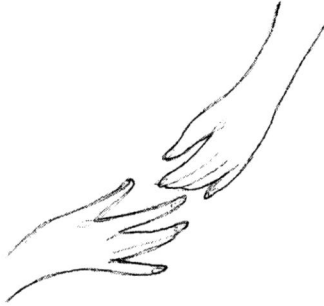

The Truth

Got the truth
You don't go far
Can't go far without
People telling the truth.
When people get the truth they don't like it
Don't like truth
That's truth and they don't like it
That's right
They know what I say
I put truth
They don't like truth
Only like to listen to lies
No truth, honesty
But there's nothing they do
What they think is true, they go
Leave it, as that

Don't Do It If You Don't Get Paid For It

If I write anything down, it goes upside down!
That's what I miss, not being able to write properly.
It's all muddle when I look at it.
Must be the brain not working properly.
I can't remember things properly.
That's part of dementia, innit?
Don't think there's much they can do about it at this age.
Might be easier if you're younger.
Supposed to be able to do something about it.
They keep talking about it.
Yeah – they do.

These People

I'll be positive
We're all the same
I got common sense
It's tough for everybody, hit the nutshell
This one's an ordinary person, got tact and
This bloke thinks he's in a memory dance
We're all the same
Be positive

Birds

Look there
She's come back again
Like one of those nosey people
Flying in and out.
There's another one to take her arm
Likes to know all your business.
Look at the wall - she's back
Ooh she's nosey, they come
Have a nose round
Go and come again.

Get on your nerves,
They wait 'til you're there
They come to your house and
See if you're alright or all wrong.
She is a mixer, a mixermighter.
They've got their dinner and
Nothing to do, just
Nose, nose around
Nosey.

I go mad, nosey bastards, swearing
All the time -
If I see her in the street I will say
'Keep away from me
You nosey old cow' -
Wants to know if you've been to bed
Been to bed
Wants to know if you've had dinner
Had dinner.
They fly in and out
All they do is look -
Come and watch you –
And tell tales.

Witness

I don't know what will happen
To the other one if I don't give in
There's no one else to take over
Not as far as we know darling
Who can I believe in?

You're a witness to what it was
Shall I write in I love you darling?
All we do is love each other

Won't Go Away

Well the world into a dangerous place now
Too many violence
Not even government able to control -
Because this thing
You know I have it
You know it won't go way
What is it?

The dementia rob all me earnings
I gave up my flat
One million people have same complaint
They reckon
(And people working in this department have it -
They come to do medication, then come back
"Lost key")

It has no friends
It attaches anybody
I heard it on the radio
They reckon
One million people have it
And it must increase
What you call it?
Dimensions?
Life is what you make

Well – It's Possible

They haven't by any chance got some hidden
receivers here?
Every second chair or something is being recorded?
Whoever is listening?
People if interested in persons' behaviour would
like to see them
Whether they do something useful or just going to
the toilet
The whole world is probably under observation by
something else
And you may be the only one writing a book about
these things
And the others observing might put into print of
their own
Completely different but at the same time
Well, it's possible

Discontented

Forgetting what they call it
Discontented?
Something like that
Unusual
In other words, it's not right

They did use a word
But I can't remember

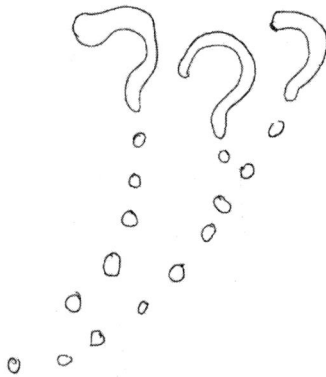

HOME

'Everybody live long in here'

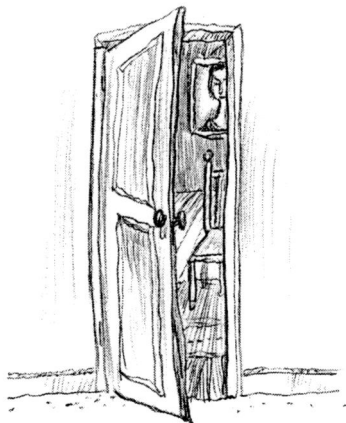

Here A Long Time

I live in the house and live good
Some time ago we have
Somewhere, family near me.

Everybody live here together
All living important to NHS
When you sick, you're sick
You see, everybody leave you

Up here a long time, long ago
Don't know which day is it
Here a long time
You come in and you lead with your heart
More hope here
Everybody live long in here
Every one

Number 65

This chair – it's so dirty feeling
I'm not in a running order
Where do you go to when you
Go out?
I keep out of walking mode
With the mainframe
In the convoy – don't go around much
I wish
Wish I could drive in a big car
Drive away in a car, oh
Oh I, I wish, wish I could
Fly just fly right away
To number 65 – Not
Drifting along at nothing

You

There are some days you are fully a tom
Other days you are just half a tom and going
Off - because you're not always together.

We have different things
But we still meet and see other people.

But mostly, you're going home
To you

Lightness

Have you got enough light?
Outside there's no light? Outside my room?
I thought there was light
Let's have more light, I love light
Do you like light?
You don't like darkness, like light
Always plenty lightness

Let's put the telly on, it gives more light
Now we've got this light and this and
Have we got enough?

There's some light in the cupboard as well
Even my family can't understand
How much I love light
Look how lovely it is outside

Can You Feel A Draft?

Everybody's here, running about
Left to right, right to left
Up the spout, through the dimple

I'm trying to read the timber
Because it tells me when the time is
I can see properly, can't see the time
Everybody's mouthing the same

How I Am

It's funny how you can go to a room
And leave yourself
I feel like I'm going a bit mental
Terrible
I can't even remember me own people
When I'm talking to them
That's how I am
That is right
Nice to be able to talk

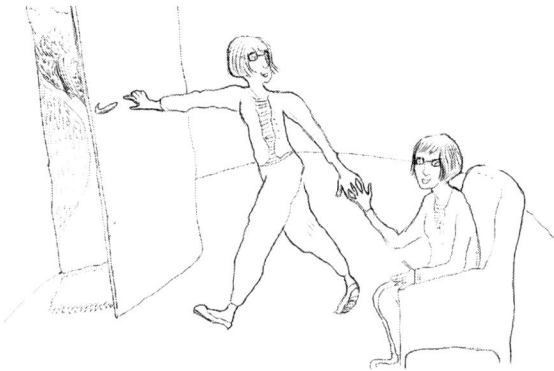

Holiday

To be allowed to go home
Even for a week and come back again
I don't want full glory
Want some satisfaction
Don't think I'm asking for the world
Not a liberty taker
A holiday to get out of here
Not a place I feel as fresh -
Shouldn't be here
It becomes monotonous
Not the place for me
Not suitable for this type of job
Not saying for life - for a holiday

Protected – A Story

What is the disease when you're imaginative?
Well I've done it.
Thought I walked from here
To Ireland and I was
Protected, knew I was
Protected in the dark:

When I got to the railway
It was a great big carriageway
Big traffic, like main buses
This way and that and when I
Heard these songs from Ireland

I realised 'But this is England!'
I felt 'How could I walk to Ireland?'
But my desire was home
And that is home I walked to
Off in this big green.

I could walk on water,
Cement like a gymnasium
Up above there were shelves
And busts and they were watching
Somehow.

I had a hat and linen boots

I put my leg over the well, a big well
There was a black hole,
I'd passed over dozens of them
Black holes all over
And cats in between.

And they and the black holes parted
And there was activity and music
At this big green, a public place
I was trying to get out
The green was danger -
I knew it would come alright,
When I paused people blessed themselves,

I was carrying a bag
Obviously heading for Ireland
I would put my boot over the edge
A black drop
And I would lever my boot
Over the edge.

And I just touched the cats
And passed buildings
Lovely music playing

No humans at all but the cats
Were dancing, in rotation
Showing me the way

I was very happy.
All lining the way, I knew
Wherever I went they would be
With me. Then I ran out of cats
Near the edge of the railway,
They had no eyes, I walked back
They weren't cats –
Pieces of wood shaped like cats
'Who put them there?'
I wasn't scared
I knew I was protected -
A wood, trees cut
To the shape of cats,

When I got to the open space
I heard an Irish voice 'She has
Cats with her, one cat, two cats...'
Just a log of wood cut beautifully
And an Irish woman's voice 'She has a black skirt'

This is what I feel about God

I know he'll lift me from here
Raise me up and out of
All the darkness

This voice was my sister

I absolutely know this is another world
Why would I leave Maida Vale
Cross so many dangerous dykes?
The singing was caring
This music was my sister
And she knew me, she said
'God save us and bless us'
And I was at home.

So I don't know if I walked
Or all was my imagination.
And I thought afterwards -
It would make a marvellous book
Because it is fear and love

At home I was fed -
And I thought of you when I was in it
Helped me get over my fear
I wouldn't go near the windows
I came home and forgot all about it

And I wake up thinking I was in Ireland -
This green place. My sister took me in.
Ireland.

Untitled

I don't know what
I'm doing here.
Wasting my time.
Sitting on my bum.
Doing nothing.
If I was at home
They'd say
'Do the washing up'

Home

I've got some new accommodation
Not very satisfying
It doesn't cure the whole
I'm the stupid one in the family
Trying to keep the flag flying
It is flying – still

I was living in a flat
Now I don't know where I am
Supposed to be living in a hotel
A terrible muddle
Can't remember things

Can't see myself living in that hotel
Doesn't make sense to me
Difficult to get back here – in my mind
I don't believe it
I don't recognise it
It doesn't feel right
There's nothing in this room to tell me what to
think is there?

Guyana

Feel lonely
Especially with my brother not here
When me brother near me
My feet on solid ground

Big family
Scattered here and there
Only me and my brother remain
I'm the big one
Carry the bulk on my shoulder
He copies everything I do
Try to better me

I am a bit separated
Too much alone for me to take it
Once I get there, feel much more comfortable

Like This

These people, some of them can't talk
And I don't know what it is, what's wrong
You see none of them talk to you
Naturally some of them cannot talk

I'd like to go somewhere strange
By myself. Have a little flat,
Had my little bungalow
Never been used to anything like this
I had my own little flat, my own little place
Then they put me in here, said
'You weren't capable of looking after your place'
I said 'I've been used to people in my own house'
You see they don't know what it's like
When it's like this do they?
When it's nothing

Him Gone Up

I didn't know people can
Just die
He the next person dead here
Old man die up to now
Just a lickle draft
Just a lickle cold
Him gone
Him gone up
Him gone to his home
People live long
He don't look like him gone

Feels Like

Go home?
Can I go home ?
A home
London
Please?
My life feels
It feels like
Misadventure
Now

OTHER

'Hope is one of our hopes'

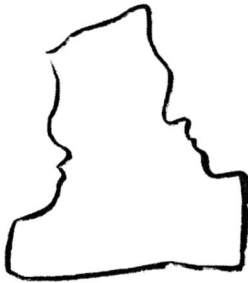

Wish Full!

We're funny creatures
Not of our doing though
Of the creators:
If there is something like a creator
I wonder what he does
And why I think of him.
In a way we refer to him
In our minds, we think he
Guides us, part of us.
Nice to know there is someone
Behind you, knows and understands
But is that wishful thinking?
Will it materialise?
Having a daydream

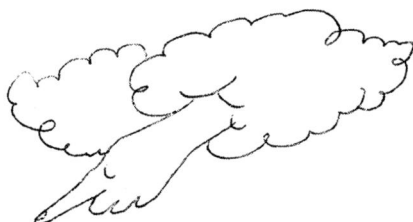

Free

You had enough?
I've had enough in here
Of everything
I'm released and pretend
Sit here, free
All free
What I like -
Quiet
All easy

This Is News

I've got burdens and things
Things that are question marks

When they begin
To start off they put all their
Wits away, in the
Bottom drawer
Have they told you anything about you?
I don't know where it goes
This all here is an old school
I'm getting a bit too big
As you grow up you have
So much to say, telling
People 'This is news'

I was confused
Everything was all packed up
And plopped over with
Fed up, low
You know
I know I've got a lot more
Things to think about
I'll tell you what
I really want to do

But I don't know the blues as much as
I know the reds – Don't know
If I'm right or wrong
Don't know if it matter much

The Whole Loving Word

Give me some of the words then!
Not bad, so many say what you want
The line, the whole:
Loving - There is loving, that is loving
This word here is loving, loving this woman
L. O. V. I. N. G - that's what I said
Love. Love. Loving word.
Have to think but I just can't -
It's only loving when it's far out
'cause it's stretching
Loving all the time
I want it full, keep it with you. Love

All You Got

All come out fresh
Today
Just for one day
You give all you've got and
You can't give no more

Mustn't grumble
You know
Things here got to –
Got to do this, do that –
But that's what's got to
Happen
You've got to sacrifice

Hope and Materialising

The whole life is a mystery
Keep hoping
Hope is a wishful thinking
I think differently to other people
One doesn't know how you feel
Can only hope

Hope is one of our hopes
That we hope
Is going to happen to us
In one way or another because
That hope we have in our mind and body
Beneficial to us all

We can only guess, by guessing
Force things to
Materialise somehow.
One doesn't know what people think
Every person is individual

Whatever we see as seeing
We don't actually but
We hope we are seeing in
The whole life

Up In The Stars

I like the feel of myself and then I feel there*
That wait or what?
Like half of it
I want to do it
But then I get
'Hup'
It's physical
And then you're ... It's like it's running away
It makes me frightened
I get myself up in the stars, it serves
Seeing what you are running
Feeling – when you go out you want to use the person
And then I feel in there, all over, no, only the beginning
Feels terrible, dirt and black but then
I'm a strainer, that's the best thing
Always be the way I think
Have you got the same?

God Deliver

You see if he got money
In his pocket he give it
God deliver, oh yes, he give it
That's why I come in here.

So a demon will come and
Fill with fear and then what?
Evil.
God deliver because heroes
Is all taken.

Everlasting

Is that you? – Everlasting
What is everlasting?
I know what you are
I'm kind of you
You think of me
I think
You haven't seen it
Everlasting
Is this everlasting?
I am a parent
I have servants
I am looking for the parent
It is hard
They are everlasting
It's gone out
It's gone out
You will see me again
I am kind of you

Feel

Everything I consider with
So it's okay. I think I –
I feel great, I feel grace
I do feel a lot – God or
Whatever it is, I feel
Great and greatness

☆

MEMORY

'All of a sudden there was nothing'

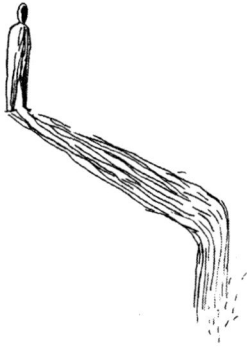

Into Words

We lost a lot of nice things, all kinds -
They go away. A little bit I got here and then
All of a sudden there was nothing I could tell you.
Could not put two together. I had a lovely story
But it took my - you know, when I found out
I couldn't talk mouth ways, like now,
I can't think.

This Tribe

Might not do much today
Poor things
The big lady there, she seems to "please, please, please"
We're retired, she's been retired
All my senior life
A long, long, long, long
What are we here?
I don't remember, I can't remember
Must be some one
I think that's the kind of person
But they don't say anything
From this tribe
I'm trying to remember
What I was doing
I said 'Get myself going'
I think I'm a poor old whiskey

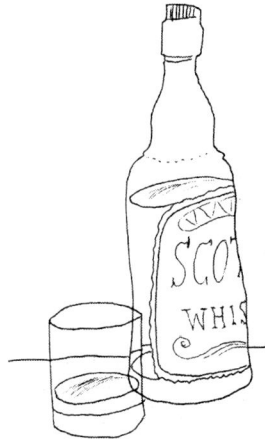

Comments On Memory

You know when you are of a certain age and
You think back of your young years
20, 30, 40 years young and you think
What would I have thought then?
The same as I would today?
We must be changing every day.
My memory has been a difficulty
When the young children try to
Remember things it's not so
Difficult for them, well it's
How shall I explain it?
The more you try to remember
The less you do
If you try to remember
And you don't
Then that's it!

Listening With Your Ears

There was one little girl:
She wasn't a naughty girl but she listened
She listened to everything she heard
And instead of ignoring her completely
Expecting her to remember eventually

Take Your Time

I know a whole –
I don't know what,
What was that now?
My problem is I have
A sister that's –
No, slow down
God bless it
My memory's bad
I get funny now
I had it all and now
Can't do a thing about –
I've got a lot of worries
Not a lot of words
You might be gone
And I'll think of it
That's how it is

Did I Do It Deliberately?

I don't want to talk about boxing
Don't want to talk.
It's heartbreaking.
The point is
All the talk and all
It boils down and ends up
Bad as the old breakdowns

After all's said and done
Everybody's said and gone
I'll still be able.

Got in a right state
Don't feel it's let me forget
Deliberately
 – Forget dates –
Did I do it deliberately?

Forgotten

Don't remember
One is in the habit of forgetting things a lot
You see, getting in to my mind
It's amazing
Sometimes can talk about things and jump
From subject and throws up questions
Should ask this, ask that
Did I ask what I'd forgotten to ask?
There's a wiggle and there's a waggle
How could one describe the difference between the two?

I Had A Great Memory

People would say
Better write this or that
I'd say no, I'll remember
And all of a sudden –
Gone, I couldn't be relied on
No way, no. If someone said
I saw 'A' and she said
So and so and so, I wouldn't know

As Far As I Know

I've got a lot going on in my mind
At the moment -
My father died you see
But I still love him – special to me
Don't think he has died
The world is too good
My father too special
Rock and roll dad!

A lot going round my mind
Sometimes I get mixed up, like mine
Many people in this world that think
About my dad, but he's gone now
He had a good memory
He looked after me
If I was doing right or wrong
He told me.
He was the one - give me lots of love

☆

DEATH

'When he take, me can't tell you'

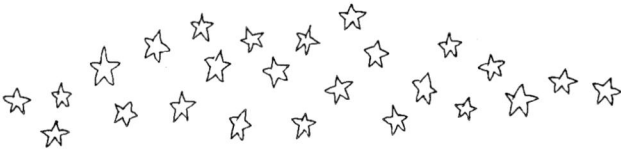

Rhythm

I'm waiting for death and it's interesting this
Waiting
For this.

National Health gave me everything
(Even a lady to talk with)
Like to finish as soon as I can

It's funny pretending
But I don't believe in anything after death
Try not to be believer
It's easier
Try the material explanation
But in the
End
There is something I can know and touch –
So,
Inside of me there is
The mass
The old, old, old education
I don't remember the music,
The letter, but I used to

If I was born Chinese
Believing in Confucianism
Be different.

More and more
For me
God is just the rhythm of the world

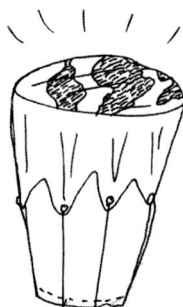

I'm Normal Man

I never kill a man
I don't have a gun
Murder is murder
I am telling you
I don't know murder
I'm normal

Feel badly, like a criminal
I know I'm not
Never done a crime in me life
Not this sort of crime
No nothing, no harm

I can tell you now I'm going to die
This talk of jail makes me sick
The truth is right, now it is truth
This murdering your life
I can feel it

When

What I tell him, I tell you
Look like mad men
And you come back
And I didn't go to church.

Church day
When your God is smiling
'You have to get things to me
Ask for forgiving, whatever you
Feeling I give.'
If the journeyman comes
You have to take the lake
When he take, me can't tell you

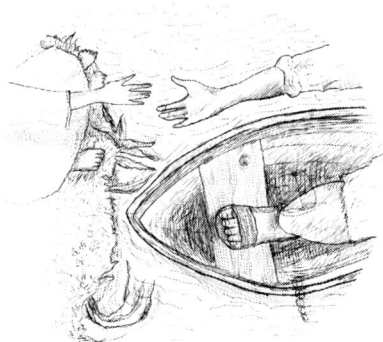

Walk

I walk at times and I walk to go
And nobody knows
I walk and walk
'Thank you God'

I'd rather just walk out to find
Nothing and nobody
There for me
I've nothing of myself
All I can do is walk

I feel I just want to walk
Into nothing sometimes

True

That's my life, my life, my life
My loves, my loves, my loves
My laughs - always laughing and joking
Loved children and now I am nothing
Just a nothing with nothing
I've forgotten my words

I'm at the end of my life
That's what it is
So real, so true, yes.

Untitled

They found him, told us we're going
We want to
Oh mummy, mum and dad with me
I will leave here and you will help me
We're old, died now mate
He loved them all
That boy he did, alone
I lay here the whole day
Will hope, hope

Find A Way Round

It's nice to see you
Feeling the words, nice
You've still got me
We'll get over it
Not gonna be the end
Of the world is it?

Thank God -
It'll go away soon
You can't live forever
No you can't
Not if you're different
I wanna enjoy it

'Cause you can't have everything
Nobody can
It's very difficult -
Still find a way round

Live Tomorrow?

I'm alright but I get depressed
Got all nice people around me
Wouldn't mind if I died right now
I just sit here and behave myself
And do what everybody else does
Don't know what I gotta do
I'll be truthful – I love you but
I wish I was dead, be pleased to die
What else can I say except
I'm proud to have you with me
I feel good and that's the truth
Will I live tomorrow or die tonight?

The Troublemakers

When you get older you
Get past all that young one
It's not great, it's horrible
Feel really sad for all this
You and I say the nicest
Sentences to each other
Love

What can we call ourselves?
The worst wishes
The troublemakers
The pensioneers

We can do without
To take up our peace
Wait - It'll pass over
Before you realise

We're hardly to become
I want to leave them until worn over
Will only be here for a while
Won't be here for a long

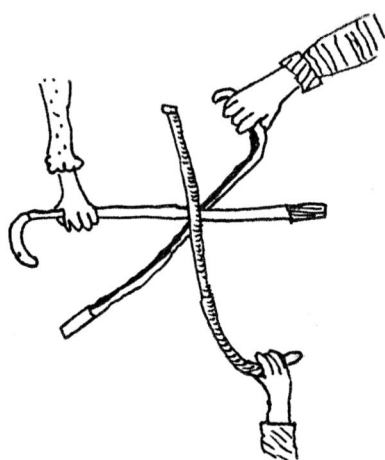

LIFE

'With bursts of happiness here and there'

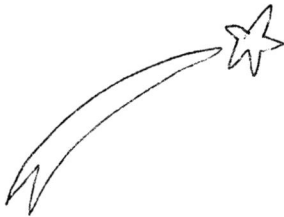

My Natural Vision Of Life Entirely

Human beings get bored
That's the way it goes
That is human
You can't explain why
Life is enigmatic

If you have a candle and
Don't take care – the light
Goes off

Life is not to be wasted
Like a packet of food
If the same all the time
Become dull
Human beings don't take it
Seriously –
Cover it up

At all life – express yourself
You have to
Gives you character
Makes it more interesting:
People, listen
Keep alert
This is human
From the bottom of my heart
Humanity – it can be heaven
It can be hell
Express yourself

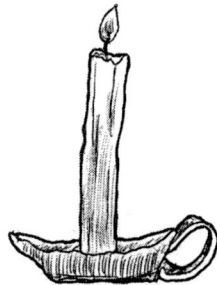

Sensitive Reaction

I haven't much of adventure / invention
Try to get myself in to conversation
Yes I must indeed yes
The poor – agree the position they are in
Can protect themselves
All depends on
Authority
If you're in power it's terrible
You can play games
Take some of that power in to the game
It's up to you whether you want to be Alive,
Regarded, In, or Rejected
You can take your
Choice
You look back
You don't even look back
You feel it –
Your whole life
You protect yourself for the federation of human life
People
It's cultural init
Important
You get inside and if you enter in to it
The front is open
Emancipation
Possibilities
You need the code word
Now and again
Don't give up
Because it could be good
Could survive
It's actually, leaving the gate open

Life Really

I've had all babies
Look how many children I've had
Seven I think, was it?
I don't know, can't remember
More, yeah, seven children
'Course that wasn't what stood
For everything

Normal

Me body's alright
I'm not sick
But I'm caught up in it
Normal
You don't have that
Me have it
You a good woman
See the body, not the fool

What Do We Do With Our Lives?

You think you've made it and then
Something comes up otherwise,
That's life - One problem after another
With bursts of happiness here and there

Life is - loads of experience
All the time. I'm a nobody -
The world seems full of nobodies!
Some stay with you forever
Others come and go

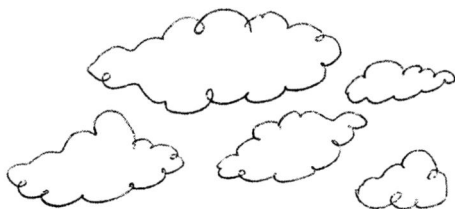

It's Alright Now, My Life

It's derry batch
Some make sense
It's why I speak
Swistory -
Wife, wife, wife
Where is she? -
Swistory
Probably here
Where am I?
What is there?
What a day!

Lived A Life

Nobody here asks what you did
In your life
It seems they seem to think
We were put on earth with broken legs
And have come for sympathy

Nobody wants to listen
I've had a stroke
Words don't come out
And they say 'Yes, yes' -
Don't really want to know

It sounds silly
But it's quite true

We have all lived a life

The Two Gaiety Girls

We always wanted to be jaunty
We have days now and again
Something pops up
We're just as we are dear
And we keep it up
As they are, lovely -
We all got our own things in here
We all get on – like a bit of happy
Happiness, games, gains
Going out, that's the joy, jaunty
Plenty of fresh air –
You and me

Human

Life Is Funny

Not so much here
Or anywhere.
Not how it used to be.
I don't know
What I am doing here,
Wasting your time.
I'm not working,
I'm not doing cooking.
Life was better
When we were younger.
Everything was younger then
Life is funny.

See? Life

Well, that's okay, that's it –
Life is entertaining and now
They are encouraging
I feel great.

Life is entertaining and so on
Well, I mean –
The life giving is the same
Been given to an older character –
Well, so it is fact

Life becomes interesting
Hear that girl?
Who isn't entertained by that?
It's all part of the stuff of life
That girl, just now, talking
It's almost that this life
The various parts of life are –
See! – Yeah,
Whatsoever and who
Comes to entertain in life
Well that's it, that's right
Feel satisfaction

A Good Idea

It's all temperamental
We get our voices through
I'm feeling very fed up
All the world is collapsing around me
Feel rather deserted
Not a good moment for me
Perhaps I'll get killed
Then I'll be out of the way

I'm being philosophical
It's a very bad moment
I don't think I live up to my reputation
It's quite good – my reputation
Think I'm basically a wastrel
Perhaps I'm not, curious isn't it?
It's all a step in the dark

The world has deserted me
So you see you've got me at a bad moment
The world doesn't take any notice
And I don't know I should expect them to
Not feeling aggrieved, just - life is difficult
Extraordinary things one goes through
I know nothing - It's all temperamental

Oh Life!

You only have one life, one life
Make the best of it dear

Sometimes I think I'm getting better
But it doesn't last - gone again
I told my doctor, thought I was mental
Still do, still do – my head is gone

You have one life dear, make the best
Get better, then goes

Life

Life goes on
And in
It all goes in
Today
It's all sort of new
Today
You live it as daily life
Forward
Seeing how it all
Turns out
At the moment, you can
Only say
I'm Learning:
Making Time
(You've got to get it down to
A Fine Art)
You make room for it
People rushing, they're unhappy
Instead of being happy
I'm probably a bit different to
Everyone else
Can't think
Straight but
Things happen sometimes
Out of the
Blue
Sometimes, the best things
Yes,
Life goes on
And in /
The ups and downs
The ins and outs

SPEAKING

'Pretend you have all the time in the world'

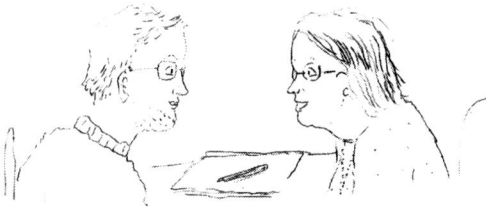

Words

I'm a worrier by nature
Can't help it
Like to have things running round
But you have to stop
Can't put in to words
That's the thing I don't like
It starts off – letters, words, then you think,
Then gets complicated
Got to work it out
Bring it down to earth
Get it on an even keel
People interfere and you're
Stumped
For
Words

We Might Be Wonderful Preachers One Day

They weren't really my words
Just came at me
Didn't plan them.
My words often do that
They come
At you and
You put them down.

I could write tons
Like thinking of things
People never think about
It suddenly comes to me
And I say things I never thought before
The right things

We might be wonderful
Preachers eventually
I always say what I think

Speaking

This place is mad, it is
I think, think it's good
To get out, I'm speaking
Look at round there
They're wanting me now
A mad one, near
Don't say much
It will come
The lost word

Comments On Language And Words

Sometimes you don't feel on top
You think I wish something like this or that happened
Could remember better
The whole life is a mystery
We can assume what we can assume
But we can't
Force it to happen.

Every year that you are
Growing up
Puts different words in to your mind
We are changing
For the worse or the better

Sometimes you don't feel on top
Point is: when you are talking about one thing
Your mind is going different directions
Sometimes use words - weren't intentional -
They fit.

We got to be a goldmine practically of words
Can stir something else up
Think, wish, remember?

All Of A Sudden

I know I'm being funny -
No one to talk to,
They nod,
I mean – here, see, look -
You hear people like that,
They come in
All of a sudden.
That's why I don't talk –
You can tell they don't really
Want to talk to you
I know I'm getting funny
She never looks at anybody

Learning

I like English but I don't speak it
Should be better off than I am
If I was educated be better off
I know that because I dream
Of education, I like it
All my brother and sisters all are
Very intelligent people
One of my brothers was
A boxer, very good boxer
One a cricketer and sportsman
Very good
My weakness was the girls
Never mind about education

I regret that now, did
The best I could, should
Have done better
Not being tough on myself
Being straight

King Or Queen

It's called 'Patient Condition'
You must not just say
'Good morning', 'Goodbye'
It minimizes the relationship
Try and appraise, interest
Tenderness, consciousness, confidence
The fact you are sharing with them
Uplift the feeling
'Feel better already',
Make us feel human
Not just a dummy.
Pretend you have all the time
In the world
We will feel like King or Queen

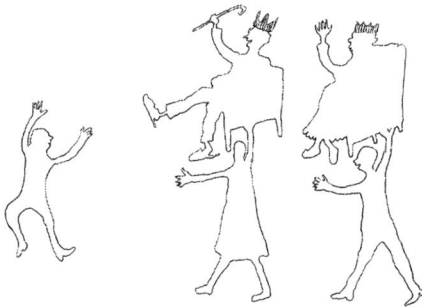

Involved

The strength
The idea,
If you don't have the part -
Catch
Tongue.
Often think it's strange,
I don't make up these words,
You came to me
When a person belonged
And then
Dropped off a bit
You can't stand to the next.
Give a lot of missing things,
It's interesting.
One becomes a little more
Alive -
It's necessary attention,
Not just there hanging -
Must come up, involved

Sense

It's sad you've got so het up about it
It's just part of your life that is gone
Taken away something precious to you
Such an important part of your life
To have conversation, be able to talk
Sense, when you haven't got any left.
Whatever happens to it I don't know
And you haven't got any, any more

Fact: It's True

I don't know what to say
Yep
I'm making a statement

Potty

I think we're all mad, it's exciting isn't it?
Would be dull as dishwater otherwise
'We're all potty' my friend said yesterday
'Yes, but isn't it exciting' I said
I mean, we're not dull
'cause I'm potty -
We were nattering away and she said
'You know I like coming to see you
Because we talk' -
She's as potty as me

I'll Tell You The Problem

I'm alright today, I've been stronger
I'm pinned in, growing smaller and
Smaller - Talk to my head, please talk
There's a body here, pains or something

I'm sitting here today, I'm saying to you
I'm going to do something -
I can see you, it's me, I drowned
This is hard, must be straight now
Perhaps that's the way, bastards
God's peace, it really is

Straight

Maaaad, I have a birdie nature
I can, I'm talking and so
It's coming up the spout
You're like me
I get to turn the page
How many are we on?
Might like when you
Finish and share, yeah
The tree is leave, branch, patient
The words – that's all mine
I might know
You're mad, but alright
Nothing is at home
And that's all straight

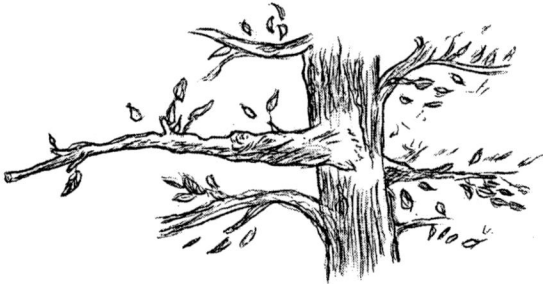

Some People

Omm imm imm
When stuff comes out all
Looolaaalodo
It all comes out
Doo doo doo
Very very very nice:
You can go up in the world
Get it, get it, get it
Some people are different
Yes.
Now.

☆

Thanks

We would like to thank the following organisations and individuals:

All the staff at all of the care homes where residencies have taken place; Guy's and St Thomas' Charity; Westminster Arts; NHS Westminster; English PEN; European Commission; Notting Hill Housing Trust; Care UK; the trustees of Living Words; Julia Miranda; Brioni Gallagher; Philip Cowell; Janet de Vigne; Tom Bishop; Elizabeth Searle; Joyce Ferguson; Ariane Koek; Nikita Lalwani; Maureen and John Howard; Myra Barrs; Krish Majumdar; Zbigniew Kotkiewicz; Paul M. Camic; Andrew Motion; Meera Syal; and Lynda Bellingham.

Lightning Source UK Ltd.
Milton Keynes UK
UKOW01f1930290616

277357UK00001B/2/P